HOW TO EFFECTIVELY CURE CHRONIC WORK-RELATED STRESS

STOP STRESSING YOURSELF AT WORK, REMOVE
ACUTE ANXIETY FROM YOUR LIFE QUICKLY,
DEVELOP A POSITIVE ATTITUDE

Jorge O. Chiesa

Table of Contents

Introduction..4

Ending Stress..5

The reasons for stress at work.............................8

How to delegate?...12

Nature in your office..15

Take a break. 17

Eliminates stressful noise 20

Decontaminate your surroundings................................22

Define priorities..25

Exercises at work..28

Conclusion: Benefits of Reducing Work-related
Stress 31

Introduction

Although stress is part of any work-related issue, excessive stress is not part of it. When you are stressed, you are not only a magnet for all kinds of "diseases," but you also invoke responsibility and ineffectiveness. This is because, when you are physically and emotionally unbalanced, your ability to deal with things is less effective and your resistance to disease is also low. Get all the information you need here.

When you feel that you are too stressed, make an effort to save yourself from total destruction and find ways to alleviate your current condition. It's your decision that can make things better for you. Why am I saying this? Because like it or not, things will get worse in the next few days.

Ending Stress

The question is, how are you going to eliminate stress at work? There are many ways to reduce stress and most of them use a personal level of focus. Here are some useful guidelines.

Organize your task according to its importance and time. There are tasks that are very important but would give you enough time to exercise. Therefore, it should be listed next to the urgent and important. Once you have finished categorizing, create a plan with a timeline and be sure to include a REST TIME and a FREE DAY in it.

Do not use your rest time to complete an incomplete task. The rest time is for your mind and body to rest. This will allow you to rest your brain and nerves, as well as your body from the stress caused by too much work. Remember, you are responsible for keeping your physical and emotional health in good shape.

Don't ignore any signs of fatigue because it could lead to a more serious problem. If you feel too tired, rest. If you feel depressed, anxious, and irritable, go ahead and rest. If you can't concentrate on what you're doing and you're losing interest in it, rest easy. If you are using alcohol and drugs to deal with stress, stop and reflect. You've already reached the limit. Don't let yourself get that far.

Strive to reduce your work stress by taking good care of yourself. You can begin to restore your physical and emotional health. Once these two are properly addressed, it will be easier for you to address your other needs, as you will feel more optimistic and strong when you feel better inside and out.

Once you are more physically and emotionally stable, your next step in getting rid of job stress is to organize and prioritize things. Make an effort to organize things first and then prioritize them. Once you have done this, you will be more guided and will regain control over things. This way you can manage stress well with self-control and confidence.

The reasons for stress at work

Employees and company owners have their own share of stress at work. Employees have different levels of stress compared to business owners because they don't have many important responsibilities like the company owner. Therefore, we cannot say that only the grassroots can experience stress because in the big picture, owners and managers also have their own struggles.

The following are the most notable causes of job stress that employees and managers should be aware of.

1. The main cause of stress is overwork. Even the most outstanding employee will definitely feel pressured when bombarded with work for a very limited period of time. Although this is irrational, it happens all the time.

2. On the contrary, there are also employees who will feel stressed when they are given less responsibility, especially when they see around them cases of layoffs and dismissals. Apparently, they don't want to be caught doing nothing, as they may be the next candidate to be fired.

3. The threat of losing a job is one of the main causes of stress at work. With the current state of our economy, job security is not constant. Sometimes layoffs are made largely while hiring has just ended.

4. Promotion is also one of the causes of stress at work. In most cases, employees are usually bored with their daily work and therefore would like to experience more challenging work in order to get more compensation. However, moving to the next level can be stressful to know that it is not just one person seeking promotion, but almost all employees who are as capable as others in terms of job performance.

5. Another cause of stress at work is doing the wrong job. If you're working on something you don't know, it'll probably burn you. Above all, if you hesitate to ask for help from someone you know who can help you with your dilemma because you don't want to be perceived as incompetent, you've just doubled the stress.

6. Mismanagement can also be serious work stress. If the head of the organization cannot lead his or her team, the subordinates are likely to feel lost and aimless. This situation can leave the team wandering and stagnant.

7. A poor work environment can also be one of the reasons employees become stressed. Of course, no one feels comfortable working with broken office equipment, insufficient lighting, noisy environments, uncomfortable furniture and more.

8. No adequate support system can also be a source of stress for employees. This is because many things happen inside the office and when things get worse, someone needs to be in the way to help them solve the problem in the proper procedure.

How to delegate?

Good, effective leaders know how to delegate. You can never be effective if you do all things for yourself. Stop playing God because that's impossible. Accept the fact that no matter how bright and skillful you are, there is no way you can do everything for yourself. When you delegate, it doesn't mean you're unable to do the job. It means that you have the power to delegate because you have greater responsibilities that you cannot afford to lose.

Imagine how the Coca-Cola Company can accommodate people's growing demand if there's only one person working on it and that's the big boss. How crazy is that? Of course, the owner will delegate responsibilities to his trusted members of the board of directors and their subordinates to meet the demand for their products.

In an employee's perspective, a manager is not considered a regular employee, not because he or she is a special person, but because his or her job is to train employees and understand their needs in order to know how to motivate them to do their job effectively. To do this, the manager needs to delegate responsibilities appropriately.

Speaking of delegating responsibilities, it is imperative that you use your own judgment about things that can be delegated and things that cannot be assigned to someone else. For example, you are working on a special project that requires your specialization. Common sense would tell you that delegating your responsibilities to someone who is not an expert in your field would mean a FAULT in every way.

In addition, try not to delegate only "dirty work" all the time because it might give the impression that you are not giving importance to the capacity of your subordinates. Give them responsibilities that can awaken their interest and release their full potential from time to time.

With that in mind, delegate the things that best suit each of your subordinates. You should consider your individual strengths and weaknesses, as well as your dedication to achieving results. Once you have finished assigning tasks, be sure to give your instructions clearly using terms that everyone can understand.

Once your computer is ready to go, be sure to regularly check its performance so you can measure it. Taking control of the project and monitoring it regularly will increase your team's success rate. However, while you are monitoring, be sure to give relevant training so that your team feels more motivated to work and more confident to do its job.

Nature in your office

One way to reduce stress at work is to bring some mark of nature into the office. Seeing a single life sign can change your mood and your outlook on stressful things.

Studies show that potting plants inside your office can help reduce toxins in the air, decrease fatigue and decrease the occurrence of disease. Therefore, the cases of sick leave are drastically reduced each month.

On top of that, plants will not only add color to the boring view of your office, but they can also help increase productivity as workers are less stressed and healthy. Plants can literally reduce toxins in the body caused by radiation from computers, mobile phones, and other radiation-emitting devices. More than that, here are some of the advantages of putting some plants in your office.

✓ Helps reduce the harmful effects of computers.
✓ Absorbs air pollutants that can result in a cleaner, uncontaminated office.
✓ Eliminates bad odor.
✓ It produces more oxygen so that the body functions properly and the mind thinks more clearly.
✓ Can promote good feelings and serene thoughts.

On the other hand, adding plants to your office is not enough. You also need to plan for your proper arrangement. No matter how you would like to bring nature into your office, always remember that it is supposed to serve your purpose and not the other way around.

Take a break.

Even machines need some rest time to function properly. Research shows that employees who are not taking breaks are likely to develop serious illnesses that can cost them the savings of a lifetime. This is definitely not good considering that we all work to live, not to live to work.

Don't work too hard

In normal situations, employees prefer to work directly rather than take a break in order to meet deadlines and avoid work overloads. Most employees today can multitask, not because they want to, but because they have to. In some companies, employees are forced to work during break time to cover all the work that needs to be done because the company does not have enough staff.

What the company's directors don't

realize is that by doing that they are pushing their employees to work too hard, which will eventually result in unproductiveness caused by stress and illness. Under these conditions, it is clear that the company is not benefiting from this situation. Instead, they are losing because employee productivity is lower compared to expenses incurred for medical bills in addition to paid sick leave.

As an employee, it is your responsibility to take care of your health. No matter how hectic your schedule, take your breaks and rest. It is best to schedule a biological break per hour to breathe fresh air and walk around the office shortly before starting work again.

You can also do some stretching to eliminate back pain and cramps. These are some of the different stretches you can apply during your rest time.

✓ Slowly tilt your head from side to side.

✓ Move your hips in a circular motion. Do the same with your shoulders.

✓ Lift one leg for about 10 seconds while the other is straight. Do the same with the other leg.

✓ Stretch your arms out for a few seconds and turn the palms of your hands.

✓ Make any movement that can release your tension in a few seconds and let your body feel the pleasure.

Eliminates stressful noise

Stress can be like a cloth we use every day if we don't do something about it. No one in this crazy world can escape the dangers of stress, but everyone can avoid it one way or another. Learn how to block out stressful noise in your daily life and choose to be more positive!

It's true that when we talk about causes of stress, we can identify many things like overwork, low wages, extended work hours, family problems, romantic problems, exasperating traffic, high bills, endless deadlines, annoying co-workers, gossiping neighbors, stubborn children, depreciating bank accounts, rising mortgage interest rates, and much more.

You can minimize these stressful cases in your daily life if you know how to manage stress effectively. The key is never to leave small responsibilities unattended. You have to understand that small things when they go unnoticed will accumulate until the time when you can no longer handle most of the stress.

Try to develop the habit of avoiding delay. Do even the simplest and smallest task you have in your diary and you will notice that life is much easier that way. There's no need to hire an expert to help you deal with your stress, as they might add to your load knowing they can charge you more than you're earning. After all, if you really had to go through so much pressure in life, you would still learn something from her that would make you even wiser.

Decontaminate your surroundings

Many people, due to the desire to have a clean and peaceful workplace, try the process of decluttering, but most of the time they fail. To do this, you must first decide and know the basics of simplicity and the benefits of a clear workplace. You can start by taking small, important steps at once because not much can be accomplished when things are rushed. Here are some effective steps to get you started.

Assign a space for incoming papers. Sometimes, we lose important documents because after it is endorsed and delivered to us, we automatically leave it somewhere where we placed it for the last time. Do not place important documents or any other documents received on someone else's desk or in your car. Develop the habit of putting things in place.

Create a clutter-free zone and make it known to many to respect your rule. Discipline yourself to keep this area untidy and clean at all times. You have to understand that you are not the only person in the office, so you can expect not everyone to respect your rules. Even so, as long as you see your area free of really clean clutter, you will eventually adapt to it and become more cautious about following its rules. Once you've succeeded with a small, uncluttered space, expand your limit until you can manage your entire office.

You should plan for a decay program even once a week and make sure you follow it. When the time comes when you need to decay, get ready to discipline yourself, because it doesn't mean you're always excited about this idea. The good thing about this is that it will become your routine and sooner or later you will get used to this constructive activity.

Assign a box for things you can't let go of but can't use either. These things can be gifts that you don't need but chose to keep because of their sentimental value. Put all these things in a box and store it somewhere away from your site, but it must be protected to make sure they are not damaged.

Give the things you no longer use to charity. Apparently, there will be few things that you have collected from your organizational activity and therefore you have something to donate. Put these things in a box and give it to the charity of your choice.

Define priorities

At work, you can expect to handle several different projects at once. Therefore, in order not to overlook something, it is necessary to prioritize it. The thing is, one project is just as important as the other. How are you going to prioritize then? Don't feel overwhelmed by this situation, understand that although everything you work for is equally important, I'm sure they won't expire on the same date. Here are the steps you can take to learn how to prioritize projects.

Since this chapter is about prioritizing projects, your first step should be to list all your priorities. When you're done with your list, rank them according to their level of importance. This must be done with the exact date of the deadlines so you can be sure you will exceed the deadline. Also, be sure to update your list and do whatever it takes to check your progress.

By doing this, you will become aware of your final and unfinished tasks and will therefore be able to act accordingly. The good thing about prioritizing is that not only will it help you organize your thoughts and actions, but it will also inspire and motivate you to continue, especially when you see great progress since you started working on a project.

Now let's go into the details of creating your priority list. For you to be guided in your company, you have to have goals to achieve. How are you going to do this? You must place a specific schedule on each of the specific tasks you listed. This will help you remember even the smallest details of your project. The key is to put even the smallest detail about your project on your list so that everything is covered.

Finally, be sure to do the simplest tasks

because when you neglect small things will accumulate and eventually become a cause of delay and panic as the deadline approaches.

Exercises at work

Stress at work is inevitable. This is because you will be working with different types of people and different types of projects. Some of the work may be new to you and the worst that could happen is that you don't have a team or someone to support you because they also have their own share of undesirable workloads.

If this is happening to you right now, be sure to deal with it to save yourself from stress and collapse. There are many ways to relieve stress at work, one of which can be done immediately during office hours. I'm talking about desk exercises that can help you relieve stress on a daily basis. Here's the list.

1. Get a good back stretch. If you are already sitting in the office for several hours, take the time to bend your back sideways as it is a good midday stretch. To do this, stand at the edge of the office chair and stretch your arms just above your head and then interlock your fingers. Tilt your body to one side and then hold it before doing the same on the other side.

2. Stretch your neck by tilting your head forward and feel your neck stretched out by holding the position for a while until you feel relieved. Do this in a different direction as you wish.

3. Stretch your upper back. Do this by sitting upright with one arm placed across your body and the other hand holding your arm right between your elbow and shoulder. Cross your arms and hold this position for a few minutes. Repeat as desired.

4. Stretch your leg. Do this using a desk to get a good balance. Stand in front of your desk and bend one leg before pulling the other towards your buttocks and feel your leg stretched. Hold the position for a few moments and repeat the operation as desired.

5. Stretch hips and thighs. Use your desk to maintain good balance as you need to pull your leg up and down. Stand in front of the desk and stretch your leg back before gradually lifting the higher leg and holding it and then lowering it. Do this on both legs a few more times.

Conclusion: Benefits of Reducing Work-related Stress

Employers and employees must pay close attention to work-related problems and recognize the causes of stress in order to address health and wellness problems. There are many different causes of stress at work and it includes overtime, excessive workload, working in the wrong job, peer pressure, poor employee support and layoffs. These are just a few of the many reasons why many workers become stressed at work.

You notice that someone feels stressed when they are always anxious, depressed, underperforming, always fatigued, and often sick. If you are experiencing such symptoms or know someone who is showing some signs of stress, don't ignore it because if you do, it is very likely that you or a certain person who is suffering from too much stress will break down sooner or later.

However, there are many effective ways to combat stress. To name a few, let's start with the self-help approach. First, think about and make a list of everything that makes you feel stressed. If you think you can handle it on your own, make a progressive plan to help you take the appropriate action to gradually eliminate each reason that causes you stress.

On the other hand, if you feel you can't do it alone, don't hesitate to ask for someone else's cooperation and discuss your concerns so that you can be properly counseled. While you're solving technical problems, don't forget to take care of your health. Exercise so often to help your body cope with stress and never underestimate the power of good, adequate sleep.

There are many benefits to reducing

work-related stress in your daily life. First, it reduces poor physical and mental capacity, so it is quick to respond to any task. Second, it reduces sickness and sick leave, giving you and your employer an advantage. Third, it increases productivity at work, which will result in greater satisfaction. Fourth, it increases your promotion advantage as you become more committed to your work and responsibilities. Fifth, it decreases the employer's expenses due to medical bills and will also improve the entire welfare of the employee.

The world can be quite a stressful environment, especially in the workplace. That's why it's important to know the signs of being overloaded and stressed in order to put an end to it. No matter how many tasks you have to perform or how busy you are, if you apply some of the above techniques, you are sure to reduce your stress levels and live a happier life. No one wants to be constantly stressed, so use these tips to change your life today!

Now yes, I wish you the best in your results, and remember, everything is practical; theory without action is of no use to you. It brings everything you learn into real life.

A big hug, your friend, Jorge!

By the way, when you achieve your results little by little, I highly recommend you, if you want to improve your social skills at work, my book, on "HOW TO TAKE WELL WITH YOUR WORKING PARTNERS", is a book that I'm sure will help you a lot to relate much better with others.

Without further ado, you can find it in the Amazon search engine, like: "HOW TO TAKE YOU WELL WITH YOUR WORKING PARTNERS" or looking for my name, like: "Jorge O. Chiesa"... *Once again I wish you success in your results!*